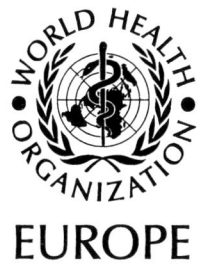

Prevention of acute drug-related mortality in prison populations during the immediate post-release period

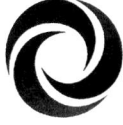

Abstract

The rate of acute drug-related mortality, or overdose deaths, among prisoners in the immediate post-release period is unacceptably high. Such incidents result from many factors, including decreased tolerance after a period of relative abstinence during imprisonment and the concurrent use of multiple drugs which, with every additional illicit drug consumed in combination with opioids, nearly doubles the risk of death from opioids. Other important factors are the lack of pre-release counselling, post-release follow-up and failure to identify those at risk. Substance dependence is a chronic disorder with high relapse rates and often requires long-term continuous treatment. There is good evidence from trials and cohort studies that opioid substitution treatment reduces the risk of overdose among opioid users.

This report identifies the main areas that need to be improved in order to decrease the risk of death. Linking prison health and public health systems closely is essential to mitigating this risk. Recommendations for preventive responses are considered across all levels of the justice system. The report includes a literature review that identifies a substantial body of research from various countries; this research supports the finding that the initial post-release period presents ex-prisoners with a significantly heightened risk of acute drug-related mortality.

Keywords

PRISONERS – statistics
SUBSTANCE-RELATED DISORDERS – mortality – prevention and control
OVERDOSE – mortality – prevention and control
DELIVERY OF HEALTH CARE – organization and administration
EUROPE

Address requests about publications of the WHO Regional Office for Europe to:
    Publications
    WHO Regional Office for Europe
    Scherfigsvej 8
    DK-2100 Copenhagen Ø, Denmark
Alternatively, complete an online request form for documentation, health information, or for permission to quote or translate, on the Regional Office web site (http://www.euro.who.int/pubrequest).

ISBN 978 92 890 4204 8

© World Health Organization 2010

All rights reserved. The Regional Office for Europe of the World Health Organization welcomes requests for permission to reproduce or translate its publications, in part or in full.

The designations employed and the presentation of the material in this publication do not imply the expression of any opinion whatsoever on the part of the World Health Organization concerning the legal status of any country, territory, city or area or of its authorities, or concerning the delimitation of its frontiers or boundaries. Dotted lines on maps represent approximate borderlines for which there may not yet be full agreement.

The mention of specific companies or of certain manufacturers' products does not imply that they are endorsed or recommended by the World Health Organization in preference to others of a similar nature that are not mentioned. Errors and omissions excepted, the names of proprietary products are distinguished by initial capital letters.

All reasonable precautions have been taken by the World Health Organization to verify the information contained in this publication. However, the published material is being distributed without warranty of any kind, either express or implied. The responsibility for the interpretation and use of the material lies with the reader. In no event shall the World Health Organization be liable for damages arising from its use. The views expressed by authors, editors, or expert groups do not necessarily represent the decisions or the stated policy of the World Health Organization.

CONTENTS

Acknowledgements _____ *iv*

Foreword _____ *v*

Recommendations to address acute drug-related mortality in prison populations in the immediate post-release period _____ *1*

    Key recommendations _____ 1

Acute drug-related mortality of people recently released from prisons: background _____ *5*

    The problem _____ 5

    The risks _____ 10

    Possible responses _____ 13

    Conclusion _____ 18

References _____ *19*

Acknowledgements

We would like acknowledge the kind assistance of Katherine Moloney, who wrote the report and made the initial draft of the recommendations during her stay at the WHO Regional Office for Europe, and to thank Regional Office staff (Alex Gatherer, Paul Hayton, Andrew Fraser, Brenda van den Bergh and Tina Kiaer) for their valuable comments.

We would also like to thank the following members of the panel for the session at the Prison Health Protection Conference in Madrid, Spain, on 29–31 October 2009 for providing very useful comments for the report: Isabelle Giraudon and Dagmar Hedrich of the European Monitoring Centre for Drugs and Drug Addiction; Michael Farrell, Professor of Addiction Psychiatry, Kings College, London; Morag McDonald of the *International Journal of Prisoner Health*; Michael Levy, Director of the Correctional Health Program at ACT Australia; and Albert Giménez, Director of the AIDS Prevention and Healthcare Programme in the Autonomous Region of Cataluña, Spain. We also thank Associate Professor Kate Dolan of the National Drug and Alcohol Research Centre, University of New South Wales, Australia, for her comments in the drafting phase.

Lars Møller
Regional Adviser a.i., Alcohol and Drugs
WHO Regional Office for Europe

Srdan Matic
Unit Head, Noncommunicable Diseases and Environment
WHO Regional Office for Europe

Foreword

Prison health is a part of public health – and for the public health system it is a challenge to give equal service to those who are hardest to reach. In general, prisoners represent a group of people with multiple health problems including drug use disorders. During incarceration they are reachable – the challenge is to make use of this unfortunate situation to the benefit of the prisoners and society.

Acknowledging this challenge, the WHO Regional Office for Europe initiated a special project on prison health back in 1995 aiming to establishing close links between prison and public health systems. In the recent years a number of guidelines, recommendations and handbooks have been published and in general the health care of prisoners has been improved.

In recent years, there has been a considerable increase in international attention to prison health. Nevertheless, the links between prison health and public health systems still need to be strengthened. An example is the clear risk of death from a drug overdose in the first weeks after release from prison. Some studies show increased risks of more than 100 times for a sex and age matched population. Most of these deaths are related to the use of illicit drugs, and most of these are accidental and therefore preventable.

A high proportion of prisoners uses drugs prior to imprisonment, and many continue in the prison setting, but more irregularly and often in a less safe way. Because of relative abstinence during imprisonment, their tolerance to drugs changes during this period. Nevertheless, the right treatment for drug dependence in prison, the right information and training, and the right follow-up after release can decrease the number of deaths.

There is evidence of interventions that help ameliorate this situation. In line with this evidence, this report provides recommendations of the best approaches to decrease the high number of deaths in the immediate post-release period.

This report is designed primarily for those in ministries who are responsible for the health of prisoners during imprisonment and after release, as well as professionals providing drug treatment and care.

The WHO Regional Office for Europe commends this book and its recommendations as a way of reducing the high post-release mortality due to overdose of illicit drugs.

Dr Nedret Emiroglu
Director a.i., Division of Health Programmes
WHO Regional Office for Europe

Recommendations to address acute drug-related mortality in prison populations in the immediate post-release period

The rate of acute drug-related mortality of prison populations in the immediate post-release period is unacceptably high. This is due to many factors, including decreased tolerance after a period of relative abstinence during imprisonment and the concurrent use of multiple drugs which, with every additional illicit drug consumed in combination with opioids, nearly doubles the risk of death from opioids. Other important factors are the lack of pre-release counselling, post-release follow-up and failure to identify those at risk.

Substance dependence is a chronic disorder with high relapse rates and often requires long-term continuous treatment. There is good evidence from trials and cohort studies that opioid substitution treatment reduces the risk of overdose among opioid users.

Key recommendations

The close linkage of prison health and public health systems is essential for success. The following recommendations should be jointly considered by both the health ministry, the ministry responsible for prison health services and the ministry responsible for prison services.

Service delivery and programmes

System-wide service delivery of drug treatment protocols and programmes for prison populations should adhere to the following principles.

Equity of care

Drug treatment provided in prison should be equal to that provided in the community. This includes staff training, therapeutic quality, coverage rates and treatment alternatives. The maintenance of homogeneity of drug treatment across prison jurisdictions and between prison and community settings is necessary to ensure therapeutic consistency.

Evidence-based practice

Opioid substitution therapy has been demonstrated to be an effective treatment option for opioid dependent persons. Opioid-dependent prisoners should be given the opportunity to commence or continue opioid substitution therapy if this is available in the community. Psychotherapeutic or psychosocial interventions and drug education are essential components of all prison drug treatment programmes.

Continuity of care and treatment stability

Due to the long persistence of substance use disorders and the severity associated with lack of treatment for this illness or therapeutic disruption, continuity of care and treatment stability are paramount. Comprehensive provision of health care services for drug-dependent prisoners is necessary throughout both the periods in the care of the criminal justice system and subsequent community reintegration. Individuals should be linked to appropriate drug or support services on first contact with the criminal justice system or when targeted as being at-risk of becoming a drug offender. The provision of services for drug-dependent people must be available while they are in police custody, pre-trial detention and prison. Furthermore, pre-release drug services are to be coordinated with and linked to appropriate after-care, to ensure uninterrupted service delivery. In so doing, substance dependent prisoners are offered sustained continuity of care.

Building partnerships and networks

Interagency partnerships between corrections-based and external service providers are essential to the establishment of effective and continuous services for prisoners. When correctly managed, the processes of government and nongovernmental agencies and community support can be integrated and coordinated, with appropriate referral systems. The importance of formal and informal community interactions, especially social support structures, are of significant importance to prisoners and provide a post-release psychological buffer.

Effective programmes depend on government officials, policy-makers, nongovernmental organizations, programme managers, researchers, prison staff and external stakeholders, as well as on the prisoners themselves and their supporters. To be effective, all interventions must address the specific post-release needs of and risks to drug dependent prisoners. Programmes need to focus on building capacity by utilizing integrated care models that incorporate psychosocial, pharmacotherapeutic and educational aspects of the best practices.

At the prison level

At the *prison level*, the service must include *building healthy therapeutic relationships*. This requires a range of needs-based, client-centred treatment modalities. Also, multifaceted team case-management partnerships are recommended. Treatment plans and service options need to be designed in consultation with service users to facilitate a culture of mutual respect, active participation, increased motivation and empowerment.

Also at this level, *education* is needed for *all stakeholders*. Prison staff, prisoners, the people that support them and external service providers (such as community care workers and nongovernmental organizations) are to be made aware of the risks of acute drug-related post-release mortality. Prisoners and the people that support them are to receive pre-release public health education in the following areas:
- drug use prevention: various methods exist to educate people about drugs, including the dissemination of information, peer support, and group or individual drug counselling;
- risk behaviour: the acute risks associated with decreased tolerance and the concurrent use of multiple drugs should be explained in detail to prisoners and the people that support them especially their families; and
- overdose prevention.

Drug-dependent prisoners and their family and community supporters are to be taught to recognize and respond to the symptoms of an overdose. The emerging evidence points towards considering teaching first aid – including the emergency use of naloxone – to those with an addiction, their social network and their family and community support. Further research in this area is urgently needed.

Moreover, at this level, *post-release vulnerability* needs to be *decreased*. To help reduce such vulnerability, holistic programmes are needed that meet the physical and/or practical and psychosocial needs of released prisoners. Prison release may represent a period of uncertainty and instability for ex-prisoners, which can increase the likelihood of drug relapse and subsequent mortality. It is necessary to ensure effective support to address the unmet:
- physical and practical needs, such as securing an accommodation and employment, managing domestic and financial affairs, and acquiring education and training in practical skills;
- psychological needs, such as deinstitutionalization, issues of traumatization and marginalization, psychiatric co-morbidity, resilience and self-esteem; and
- social needs, such as familial or community reintegration and social and parenting skills.

At the national level
At the *national level*, the provision of key structures and services must include:
- providing a comprehensive, countrywide framework of drug treatment
- determining which service or agency must take responsibility
- recognizing and addressing the specific needs of particular subgroups
- monitoring, risk assessment and evaluation of interventions.

Providing a comprehensive, countrywide framework of drug treatment
A comprehensive, countrywide framework of drug treatment needs to be incorporated into all levels of the criminal justice system. This strategy should be integrated into or consolidated with the efforts of community drug treatment within the national public health system. The main principle is that, where possible, it is preferable for individuals with a substance use disorder to be diverted to an appropriate community treatment facility rather than be sent to prison. In cases where prison is deemed necessary, drug treatment should be provided, based on formalized end-to-end strategies of throughcare and after-care.[1]

Determining which service or agency must take responsibility
Determining which service or agency must take responsibility for and address the needs of individuals at risk of acute drug-related mortality after release from prison

---

[1] Fox et al. (2005) give these definitions: "The term *'throughcare'* refers to arrangements for managing the continuity of care which begin at an offender's first point of contact with the criminal justice system through custody, court, sentence, and beyond into resettlement. *'Aftercare'* is the package of support that needs to be in place after a drug-misusing offender reaches the end of a prison-based treatment programme, completes a community sentence or leaves treatment. It is not one simple, discrete process involving only treatment but includes access to additional support for issues which may include mental health, housing, managing finance, family problems, learning new skills and employment".

requires conceptual reframing of prison health mandates to incorporate post-release well-being. This may necessitate:
- evaluating data collection, to continually monitor post-release outcomes in prison health data and so adequately identify service gaps;
- analysing the legal frameworks and extent of duty of care and accountability for the health of people after their release from prison; and
- including, under the jurisdiction of this national structure, individuals serving community sentences, on home leave and those on parole.

These processes should begin prior to release and should be integrated into drug treatment programmes to ensure holistic need-based programmes.

Recognizing and addressing the specific needs of particular subgroups
Programme design should target the assessed needs of high-risk sociodemographic subgroups, including women and foreign national people. Also, standardized risk assessment and screening are useful in identifying individual prisoners who are at an increased risk of drug-related post-release mortality and who would benefit from specialized programmes and support.

Monitoring, risk assessment and evaluation of interventions
Monitoring, risk assessment and evaluation of interventions includes the implementation of a standardized monitoring protocol to:
- determine baseline mortality rates
- assess prisoner needs, inside prison and upon release
- document implementation of interventions and the success of these measures
- identify gaps in service provision.

Also, research is important to evaluate interventions to reduce post-release mortality, and specific indicators should be developed.

Acute drug-related mortality of people recently released from prisons: background

The problem

The lifetime prevalence of illicit drug use is overrepresented among prisoners. While this rate differs extensively by country, between 2000 and 2007 the majority of surveys of incarcerated populations in the European Union and Norway documented a lifetime prevalence of over 50% (EMCDDA, 2008). In some of the countries examined, 50–60% of prisoners recalled ever having used heroin, amphetamines or cocaine, and over a third recalled ever having injected drugs. In Asia, Europe and North America, opioid-dependency is disproportionately high among prisoners, representing as much as 80% of prisoners in central Asia, while the drug of choice in Latin America is cocaine (Kastelic, Pont & Stöver, 2008). Also, considering the high turnover rate in prisons (Stöver, 2001; Møller et al., 2007), large numbers of prisoners with a history of drug use are incarcerated and then released into the community annually.

This report examines the effect of the prison experience on post-release drug-related outcomes. Specifically, it presents a literature review of the problems and the risks associated with acute drug-related mortality of prison populations in the immediate post-release period. This is followed by a discussion of possible preventive responses.

Individuals who have served a prison sentence are characterized by poorer health outcomes than individuals within the general community, with ex-prisoners having significantly raised natural and unnatural rates of mortality. Hobbs et al. (2006) conducted a data-linkage cohort study of all 13 667 prisoners in Western Australia discharged between 1995 and 2001 (a total of 26 674 discharges). Deaths due to the acute or chronic effects of drugs, injury or poisoning accounted for about three quarters of indigenous female, non-indigenous female and non-indigenous male deaths and a large proportion of prisoner excess mortality. Also, research from several countries report increased drug-related post-release mortality rates, compared with the general population: Australia (Coffey et al., 2003; Graham, 2003; Stewart et al., 2004; Kariminia et al., 2007a), Denmark (Christensen et al., 2006), England and Wales (Singleton et al., 2003; Farrell & Marsden, 2008), France (Verger et al., 2003), Scotland (Seymour, Oliver & Black, 2000; Shewan et al., 2000), Switzerland (Harding-Pink, 1990) and the United States of America (Binswanger et al., 2007).

Table 1 summarizes the findings of studies that document the drug-related standardized mortality ratios (SMRs) of ex-prisoners compared to a reference population. There is a vast disparity in SMRs between these studies. However, the data presented consistently show that post-release drug-related mortality rates greatly surpassed the adjusted rates of the respective general populations from which the prisoner cohorts were drawn. Cumulatively, the findings support the hypothesis that released prisoners are at a significantly heightened risk of drug-related death relative to other residents in the general population.

Table 1. Drug-related SMRs of ex-prisoners and a reference population

Study	SMR (95% CI) of post-release drug-related mortality	Time frame (post-release)	Reference population	SMR adjustments (original study)
Binswanger et al. (2007)	Males and females = 129.0	First 2 weeks	Residents of Washington State, USA	Age, sex and race
Christensen et al. (2006)	Males and females = 61.9 [a]	First 2 weeks	General population of Denmark	Age and gender
Farrell & Marsden (2008)	Males, first week after release = 28.3 Males, second week after release = 15.8 Females, first week after release = 68.9 Females, second week after release = 56.3	First and second weeks (calculated separately)	General population of England and Wales	Age and gender
Harding-Pink (1990)	Males and females = 50.0 [a]	First 45 days	Population of Geneva, Switzerland	Age and sex
Kariminia et al. (2007a)	Males = 14.5 Females = 50.3	Not time limited, follow-up ranged from 1 day to 15 years (median = 7.7 years)	Population of New South Wales, Australia	Age and sex
Singleton et al. (2003)	First week after release = 37.1 Second week after release = 12.4 (male and female combined) [b]	First and second weeks (calculated separately)	General population of England and Wales	Age and gender
Stewart et al. (2004)	Female Aboriginal = 3.3 Female non-Aboriginal = 115.9 Male Aboriginal = 2.9 Male non-Aboriginal = 20.1	Not time limited, follow-up ranged from 0–2160 days (median = 1223 days)	Aboriginal and non-Aboriginal populations of Western Australia aged 20–40 years	Ethnicity, age and gender
Verger et al. (2003)	15–34 years = 124.1 35–54 years = 274.2 (male only)	First year	General population of France	Age and gender

Note. SMRs are expressed relative to 1. Descriptive statistics have been standardized and data adjusted accordingly to facilitate comparison between studies.
[a] Authors' calculations: the estimate was based on deaths per 1000 person-years of reference population and discharged prisoners. No confidence interval (CI) was obtained.
[b] The CI was not specified by Singleton et al. (2003).

Also, while there is a tendency towards elevated drug-related mortality of ex-prisoners in the community, this is most salient in the immediate post-release period (EMCDDA, 2008). In a sample of 12 438 traceable prisoners discharged from prisons in England and Wales in June or December 1999, Singleton et al. (2003) established 137 deaths over the study period. Of these deaths, 79 were drug-related. Significantly, in the first week after discharge, there were 13 recorded deaths, 12 of which were attributable to drugs (representing an equivalent death rate of 50.4 deaths per 1000 ex-prisoners per year). In the following week, there were 6 deaths, 4 of them drug related (16.8 deaths per 1000 ex-prisoners per year). The mortality rate then decreased rapidly and, from week five, levelled off at about 2 deaths a week. The decline in all-cause mortality was primarily due to decreased drug-related deaths in the two-week period after release. Relative to the general population, ex-prisoners were 40.2 times more likely to die in the first week after discharge, with 92% of deaths credited to drug-related causes and 18.6 times (67% due to drugs) in the second week after discharge.

Of a retrospective Danish cohort of 15 885 registered drug users, 6 019 had at least one prison discharge during the study period, 1996–2001 (Christensen et al., 2006). During this period, 145 post-release drug-related deaths were observed (11.9 deaths per 1000 person-years), of which 24 occurred in the first 2 weeks of liberation (117.7 deaths per 1000 person-years). The latter category exceeds the mortality of the general population (1.9 deaths per 1000 person-years) by a factor of 62 and accounted for 92% of all deaths in the two-week period after release.

Similarly, a retrospective cohort analysis of 48 771 prisoners released in England and Wales between 1998 and 2000 identified 442 deaths during the study period, 59% ascribed to drugs (Farrell & Marsden, 2008). In the first week after release, male prisoners were 29.4 times more likely to die than their male counterparts in the community, and women were 68.9 times more likely to die than women in the community; 96% of male and 100% of female deaths were attributed to drugs. In the second week, this mortality ratio (and percentage attributed to drug-related causes) was 20.4 (78%) and 56.3 (100%) for male and female ex-prisoners, respectively.

A comparable data-linkage study of 30 237 ex-prisoners from the Washington State Department of Corrections, United States of America, discharged between July 1999 and December 2003, documented 443 deaths during the study period (7.8 deaths per 1000 person-years) (Binswanger et al., 2007). Of these deaths, 23% were attributed to drugs. Within the first two weeks after discharge, 27 of the 38 deaths were drug-related – that is, a death rate of 18.4 deaths per 1000 person-years. Also, during this immediate post-release period, the acute relative risk of drug-related mortality was 129 when examined against the general population. Thus, a marked elevation in mortality among ex-prisoners may be observed during the two weeks directly after release, due largely to drug-related causes. All-cause mortality then stabilizes in subsequent weeks, reflecting diminished drug-related mortality.

Discrete lifestyle factors, such as quantity of drugs used and levels of risk-taking behaviour, may be controlled by temporal matching. In this manner, the disproportionately high mortality observed within the first two weeks after release may be appraised within this high-risk population. Table 2 collates literature that examines the relative risk of drug-related ex-prisoner drug-related mortality in the first two weeks after release against a specified period thereafter.

The data presented illustrate that, in all studies, the prospect of ex-prisoners dying from drugs in the first two weeks after discharge exceeds that of drug-related death during a subsequent occasion at liberty. The mean risk of drug-related death by ex-prisoners in their first two weeks after release is 8 times that of any measured time thereafter (see Table 2). This finding supports the growing body of literature that substantiates the acute risk of drug-related mortality encountered by newly released prisoners. Significantly, the adjusted comparisons do not differ substantially, according to the time since release from which the comparison was drawn.

Furthermore, drug-related mortality in the first two weeks after release surpasses both in-prison suicides (Seaman, Brettle & Gore, 1998; Bird & Hutchinson, 2003; Kariminia et al., 2007c) and in-prison drug-related deaths (Kariminia et al., 2007c). Drug-related ex-prisoner mortality as a percentage of all-cause mortality more closely resembles drug-related deaths among prisoners serving community correctional orders, in contrast to drug-related prisoner deaths (Sattar, 2001). Significantly, individuals sentenced to post-prison parole orders have considerably larger all-cause mortality rates than prisoners serving other community supervision classifications, with drugs being the most common cause of mortality (Biles, Harding & Walker, 1999; Sattar, 2001). Released prisoners under community supervision continue to represent a neglected (but high risk) population.

Table 2. Temporal matching in studies assessing the relative risk (RR) of drug-related death in the first two weeks after release, compared with other times afterwards

Study	Country	RR (temporal matching)	Temporal comparison
Bird & Hutchinson (2003)	Scotland	7.4	Subsequent 10 weeks (3–12 weeks)
Christensen et al. (2006)	Denmark	4.6[a]	Subsequent 10 weeks (3–12 weeks)
Farrell & Marsden (2008)	England and Wales	Male = 8.3　Female = 10.6	At 52 weeks
Kariminia et al. (2007c)	Australia (New South Wales)	Male = 9.3　Female = 6.4	At 26 weeks
Seaman, Brettle & Gore (1998)	Scotland (Edinburgh)	7.7[b]	Subsequent 10 weeks (3–12 weeks)
Singleton et al. (2003)	England and Wales	First week = 12.5　Second week = 4.2	13–52 weeks

[a] Study participants: drug users.
[b] Study participants: injecting drug users infected with HIV.

Kariminia et al. (2007a) conducted the largest cohort study to date that investigated long-term cause-specific mortality of adult prisoners. The analysis consisted of a retrospective data-linkage of all 85 203 adults incarcerated in New South Wales,

Australia, from 1988 to 2002, inclusive. The investigation established 5137 deaths (4714 men, 423 women) of which drug-related mortality accounted for 31% (SMR 12.8) and 47% (SMR 50.3) in men and women, respectively. This constituted about a quarter (26%) of all drug-related deaths in New South Wales during the fifteen-year period. This figure is consistent with other studies of prisoners in Australia (Coffey et al., 2003; Graham, 2003) and Scotland (Shewan et al., 2000) that examine cohorts that differ by age and sex.

Of note, however, are the time trends in mortality rates obtained by Kariminia et al. (2007a), which depict a decline in all-cause mortality over the study period relative to the New South Wales population. This is largely attributable to reductions in drug-related deaths and suicides. The causality of this decreasing trend in drug-related mortality is yet to be established and merits further investigation. One hypothesis for this finding, which the authors present, is enhanced provision of mental health services and their availability to prison populations. Indeed, the study coincides with the endorsed expansion of methadone maintenance treatment as the principle component of Australia's harm minimization drug policy in 1985 and the introduction, in 1986, of methadone maintenance treatment in New South Wales prisons. Such treatment, as a means of harm reduction, is recognized for its protective function against premature mortality among heroin users in community settings (Gunne & Grönbladh, 1981; Langendam et al., 2001). Certainly, research from Australia, Germany, Italy, Sweden and the United States of America collectively confirm that, compared with untreated opioid-dependence, retention in methadone maintenance treatment reduces mortality by 75% (Gearing & Schweitzer, 1974; Cushman, 1977; Grönbladh, Ohlund & Gunne, 1990; Davoli et al., 1993; Poser, Koc & Ehrenreich, 1995; Caplehorn et al., 1996). Similar results have been reported in France (Auriacombe et al., 2004) with buprenorphine, a partial opioid agonist–antagonist administered as an alternative substitute medication.

With reference to prison populations, Dolan et al. (2005) evaluated all-cause mortality in a follow-up study of 382 incarcerated male participants enrolled in a randomized controlled trial of prison-based methadone maintenance treatment in New South Wales. In the four-year follow-up, retention in methadone maintenance treatment was negatively correlated with mortality. All 17 recorded deaths occurred among individuals having either never received methadone maintenance treatment or discontinued prison-based methadone maintenance treatment prior to discharge, reflecting an untreated mortality rate of 20 deaths per 1000 person-years. In contrast, prison detoxification programmes, which represent a treatment interruption in community-based substitution therapy, neither curb post-release reversion to injecting practices nor reduce drug-related mortality compared with controls (Shewan et al., 2001). Despite a relatively favourable twelve month relapse rate of 78% (12% less than comparable inpatient programmes), the Mountjoy Prison Detoxification Programme in Ireland registered high drug-related post-release mortality after completion of treatment (Crowley, 1999). As a result, Crowley advocates the provision of prison-base methadone maintenance treatment for the majority of incarcerated drug users to whom detoxification is inappropriate. In addition, prison-based methadone maintenance treatment is economically viable, as the cost entailed does not exceed that of community-based methadone maintenance treatment, and the cost per death avoided compares favourably with similar health measures (Warren et al., 2006).

The risks

Acute drug-related mortality, or overdose, is the principle cause of drug-related death among ex-prisoners immediately after release. The excess rates of acute drug-related mortality observed in the initial post-release period is thought to be a consequence of many factors. Two compounding processes represent the foremost factors for acute drug-related mortality of former prisoners immediately after liberation. These are decreased tolerance after a period of relative abstinence during imprisonment and concurrent use of multiple drugs which, with every additional illicit drug consumed in combination with opioids, nearly doubles the risk of death from opioids. Inherently interrelated with these processes are risk factors such as treated and untreated chronic disease progression and socio-demographic determinants. These factors include the lack of pre-release counselling and post-release follow-up, and failure to identify those at risk. It is therefore appropriate to examine the underlying mechanisms and risk factors that contribute to these processes.

Imprisonment frequently represents a period of decreased drug availability and a resultant abstinence or reduction in drug intake for the duration of the prison term. Lowered physiological tolerance of the pre-prison drug quantity follows this interval of relative abstinence. This places prisoners at a heightened risk of acute drug-related mortality upon resuming substance use after being released. By the same process of lowered tolerance, acute drug-related mortality is disproportionately high among ex-prisoners that relapse subsequent to prison methadone detoxification (Harding-Pink, 1990; Crowley, 1999). Indeed, having undertaken methadone detoxification within the past year is positively correlated with overdose, whereas the inverse is true of methadone maintenance (Seal et al., 2001). Thus, as noted earlier, retention in prison and community methadone maintenance treatment is associated with a decline in mortality among ex-prisoners (Dolan et al., 2005). This may be understood by appreciating that substance dependence is a chronic disorder that disposes sufferers to high relapse rates and often requires long-term continuous treatment. Substance-dependency is overrepresented among both prison populations (Fazel, Bains & Doll, 2006; Kastelic, Pont & Stöver, 2008) and ex-prisoner drug-related fatalities (Harding-Pink, 1990; Singleton et al., 2003; Farrell & Marsden, 2005).

According to non-prisoner-specific studies (see, for example, Zador, Sunjic & Darke, 1996), drug-related deaths among ex-prisoners typically occur in people older than 25 years of age (Davies & Cook, 2000; Sattar, 2001; Singleton et al., 2003; Verger et al., 2003; Binswanger et al., 2007), suggesting extended careers of substance use. Singleton et al. (2003) identified that almost three quarters (72%) of the drug-related excess mortality ratio occurred among prisoners aged 25–39 years at the time of release. In a representative survey of prisoners, Singleton et al. (2003) determined that, of the subset of prisoners who subsequently died of drug-related causes (as compared with the whole sample), 72% were assessed as being drug-dependent within the year of interview (52%), with 40% dependent on opiates and stimulants (12%); 85% used drugs in the month before their prison term (57%) and 54% had abstained from drugs while in prison (55%). Both drug use in the month before incarceration and in-prison drug abstinence were found to be independently associated with post-release drug-related mortality in the final logistic regression model. Also, re-offenders are at an increased risk of post-release death (Harding-Pink, 1990; Hobbs et al., 2006;

Kariminia et al., 2007b), which implies a cumulative detrimental effect of periods of reduced tolerance due to sporadic disruption to drug or treatment habits. Also, post-release drug-related mortality is associated with older, drug-dependent users not currently receiving maintenance pharmacotherapy and having experienced drug or treatment discontinuity as a consequence of incarceration.

In addition, what is apparent on examination of substance-related death by age at the time of release is the distinct age difference of drug-related mortality between men and women. Women consistently exhibit a younger age profile than do men. Farrell & Marsden (2005) found that over two thirds of excess drug-related mortality occurred in men aged 25–39 years of age, and women aged 20–29 years. Also, Kariminia et al. (2007b) noted that the age distribution of deaths differs by gender, such that women show a decreasing trend with age while mortality among men is prominent among the youngest and oldest age groups.

When compared with their male counterparts, female ex-prisoners represent a discrete substance-related mortality profile. While more male ex-prisoners die of post-release drug-related causes, female ex-prisoners are proportionately more at risk of dying from such causes (Graham, 2003; Steward et al., 2004; Kariminia et al., 2007a; Farrell & Marsden, 2008). This may be a function of the drug classes and combinations that women utilize. Female drug-related fatalities were more frequently associated with benzodiazepines (Harding-Pink, 1990), cocaine and tricyclic antidepressants and with more than one class of drug than were corresponding male fatalities (Farrell & Marsden, 2005). For both men and women, however, almost 90% of post-release substance-related deaths in Australia, England and Wales, and Switzerland involved opioids (Harding-Pink, 1990; Davies & Cook, 2000; Singleton et al., 2003; Farrell & Marsden, 2005). Table 3 illustrates the predominance of opioids in toxicological analyses of drug combinations in studies from Australia and Europe. Heroin or morphine was documented as both the most commonly reported drug and the principle cause of death in these studies. This is contrary to findings from the United States of America, which implicate cocaine in the majority of drug-related deaths (Binswanger et al., 2007). In the two week period post-release a greater proportion of drug-related deaths reportedly involved heroin and cocaine while less have been found to involve alcohol than during subsequent times at liberty (Farrell & Marsden, 2005; Binswanger et al., 2007).

A significant percentage of post-release drug-related deaths result from the use of multiple psychoactive substances (Harding-Pink, 1990; Davies & Cook, 2000; Seymour, Oliver & Black, 2000; Shewan et al., 2000; Singleton et al., 2003; Farrell & Marsden, 2005; Binswanger et al., 2007). According to the polydrug use theory, the respiratory depressive effects of opioids are enhanced by concurrent administration of opiates and other drugs, especially substances that act on the central nervous system (Darke & Zador, 1996). It is by this polysubstance mechanism that intake of opioids at dosages regularly tolerated may cause death. Indeed, Gossop et al. (2002) established that, for every supplementary illicit drug administered in conjunction with an opioid, the risk of death from opioids nearly doubles. Excessive alcohol consumption, when combined with illicit drugs, was also found to increase mortality. McGregor et al. (1999) reported that co-administration of heroin and psychotropic substances occurred in three quarters of fatal overdoses among ex-prisoners in the month after release. The authors reflect on the inherent difficulties in determining the

Table 3. Findings of studies on post-mortem toxicological combinations of drug-related ex-prisoner deaths by number (and percentage) of cases

Drugs or drug combinations identified	Number (and percentage) of deaths, by study and cause									
	Davies & Cook (2000)[a]	Farrell & Marsden (2008)		Harding-Pink (1990)[b]		Seymour, Oliver & Black (2000)[c]	Shewan et al. (2000)[d]		Singleton et al. (2003)	
	Drugs alone	Drugs alone	Drugs plus alcohol	Drugs alone	Drugs plus alcohol	Drugs alone	Drugs alone	Drugs plus alcohol	Drugs alone	Drugs plus alcohol
Single drugs										
Heroin/morphine	6 (13)	57 (22)	30 (12)	ND	4 (31)	10[e] (53)	ND	ND	34 (43)	7 (9)
Methadone	ND	9 (4)	2 (1)	ND	ND	1 (5)	ND	ND	4 (5)	2 (3)
Other opioid or opioid-based substances	ND	6 (2)	5 (2)	ND	ND	ND	ND	ND	3 (4)	1 (1)
Tricyclic antidepressants	ND	5 (2)	1 (0)	ND	ND	ND	ND	ND	1 (1)	ND
Other	ND	6 (2)	2 (1)	ND	ND	1 (5)	ND	ND	ND	ND
All single drug cases	6 (13)	83 (32)	40 (16)	ND	4 (31)	12 (63)	ND	ND	42 (53)	10 (13)
Multiple drugs										
More than one opioid	ND	4 (2)	4 (2)	ND	ND	1 (5)	ND	ND	2 (3)	1 (1)
Opioid(s) plus benzodiazepines	10 (22)	13 (5)	16 (6)	2 (15)	6 (46)	6 (32)	5 (50)	2 (20)	1 (1)	3 (4)
Opioid(s) plus cocaine	ND	11 (4)	6 (2)	ND	ND	ND	ND	ND	3 (4)	ND
Opioid(s) plus one other type of drug	ND	14 (5)	10 (4)	ND	ND	ND	2 (20)	ND	1 (1)	ND
Opioid(s) plus two or more other types of drugs	ND	14 (5)	9 (4)	ND	ND	ND	ND	ND	1 (1)	1 (1)
Opioid(s) plus benzodiazepines plus other types of drugs	24 (53)	6 (2)	9 (4)	1 (8)	ND	ND	1 (10)	ND	2 (3)	3 (4)
Two or more other types of drugs	ND	5 (2)	4 (2)	ND	ND	ND	ND	ND	ND	1 (1)
Unspecified mixture of drugs	5 (11)	5 (2)	3 (1)	ND	ND	ND	ND	ND	5 (6)	2 (3)
All multiple drug cases	39 (87)	72 (28)	61 (24)	3 (23)	6 (46)	7 (37)	8 (80)	2 (20)	15 (19)	11 (14)
Total cases	45 (100)	155 (61)	101 (39)	3 (23)	10 (77)	19 (100)	8 (80)	2 (20)	57 (72)[f]	21 (27)[f]

Note. ND = not determined.
[a] Unrepresentative retrospective sample of post-release female-only deaths. Alcohol was reported in 3 (7%) unspecified cases.
[b] Drug-related deaths in the first 45 days post-release.
[c] Drug-related deaths in the first 2 days post-release. The number of cases involving alcohol was not specified.
[d] Female-only drug-related deaths in the first year post-release.
[e] In one of these cases, methadone was present in the blood. However, the cause of death was pulmonary congestion and oedema.
[f] In one case, mortality was not directly linked to an episode of use.

relative effects of diminished tolerance versus the use of multiple psychoactive drugs. The cumulative effect of these distinct processes, however, places ex-prisoners at a significantly elevated risk of acute drug-related mortality in the immediate post-release period, proportional to other periods after release. Prisoners are insufficiently aware of the risks posed by either decreased tolerance or the concomitant use of multiple psychoactive substances. It is the responsibility of pre-release prison programmes to educate prisoners adequately about the nature and extent of these risks.

Besides age and gender, a number of sociodemographic characteristics are associated with an increased risk of post-release drug-related mortality. Studies from Australia, England and Wales indicate that prisoners from the dominant ethnic background are at a relatively heightened risk of drug-related mortality (Singleton et al., 2003; Stewart et al., 2004; Farrell & Marsden, 2005; Kariminia et al., 2007b). A multivariate statistical analysis found that in-prison psychiatric hospital admission (Kariminia et al., 2007b), suicidality, in-prison victimization and taking medication that acted on the central nervous system (Singleton et al., 2003) are independent predictors of drug-related mortality. However, similar analyses of criminological determinants reveal contradictory findings between studies in the measure of principle type of offence (Singleton et al., 2003; Kariminia et al., 2007b). Additional independent risk factors for post-release drug-related mortality include living off crime before the current prison term and having a primary support network of less than four people (Singleton et al., 2003). These findings emphasize that this population lacks formal and informal psychosocial support structures. It is therefore necessary to contextualise drug overdose the within the wider framework of prisoner experiences. This provides a potential avenue of redress by means of incorporating psychosocial needs-based programmes into in-prison and after-care treatment protocols.

In a similar manner, the setting of post-liberation drug-related mortality (Table 4) highlights the social obstacles encountered by ex-prisoners on release – in particular, the difficulty of procuring permanent housing (Davies & Cook, 2000). At least half of deaths occurred in temporary accommodation or in a public place. However, this too provides insight into potential target areas for programmes, such as assistance in securing accommodation. Furthermore, as a significant proportion of these drug-related deaths occurred in residential settings, observers may be trained to recognize, intervene and seek medical assistance in response to an overdose (Singleton et al., 2003; Farrell & Marsden, 2005).

Possible responses

In accordance with international law and human rights instruments, the effect of imprisonment on human rights is limited to the deprivation of liberty (United Nations, 1990), referred to as "limited exceptionalism" (Betteridge, 2005:69). As such, prisoners, like all people, are to be afforded the highest attainable standard of physical and mental health (United Nations, 1946, 1948, 1976b), fulfilling the principle of "equivalence of care" between prison and community health care service provision (United Nations, 1982, 1990; WHO, 1993; CE Committee of Ministers, 1998, 2006; UNODC, UNAIDS & WHO, 2006). Also, a consolidated system of health care in prisons is advocated, such that prison health systems interact or integrate with national public health systems (United Nations, 1955; CE Committee of Ministers, 1998; WHO Regional Office for Europe, 2003).

Table 4. Studies of the settings of post-liberation drug-related mortality, by number (and percentage) of cases for which information was available

Setting and other data	Number (and percentage) of deaths by study		
	Davies & Cook (2000)[a]	Farrell & Marsden (2005)	Singleton et al. (2003)
Permanent place of residence	10 (26)	112 (50)	13 (34)
Temporary accommodation	17 (44)		
Other's home/unspecified indoor location	ND	51 (23)	12 (32)
Hostel (local authority or probation)	ND	26 (12)	6 (16)
Public space (includes car parks, railway stations and on streets)	12 (31)	34 (15)	4 (11)
Hospital	0	0	3 (8)
Other	0	1 (0)	0
Number of cases	39 of 45 (87)	224 of 261 (86)	38 of 79 (48)
Exclusions (data unavailable)	6 cases	37 cases	41 cases

Note. ND = not determined.
[a] Unrepresentative retrospective sample of post-release female-only deaths.

As expressed by the joint WHO, United Nations Office on Drugs and Crime, and Joint United Nations Programme on HIV/AIDS position paper on substitution maintenance therapy (WHO, UNODC & UNAIDS, 2004), a flexible needs-based client-centred approach to opioid dependence is necessary to aptly address the individual needs of clients. Utilization of pharmacotherapy, of which substitution maintenance therapy is an "important component" (WHO, UNODC & UNAIDS, 2004:13), psychotherapy, psychosocial rehabilitation and risk reduction interventions are thus endorsed. With respect to prisons, harm reduction and prevention measures are recommended (WHO, 1993; WHO Regional Office for Europe, 2005); and in nations where methadone maintenance treatment is available in the community, this treatment is to be extended to prisoners, so that they may continue or initiate substitution therapy while in custody (WHO, 1993; Lines et al., 2004). Failure to do so may constitute torture or cruel, inhumane or degrading treatment or punishment, or a breach of the right to life (United Nations, 1976a, 1988).

While regional and international instruments detail comprehensive recommendations on minimum standards of prison health, it is the responsibility of national authorities to determine how to best implement these principles. Borzycki (2005) categorizes prison throughcare in terms of a three-tiered model for conceptualizing service provision within a jurisdiction. The model's tiers are:
(a) the philosophy that informs corrections, which is linked to the aims and methods that are used to achieve those aims;
(b) system-wide service delivery; and
(c) specific programmes delivered within operational frameworks.

The model states that correctional ethos informs policy, which in turn is implemented through system-wide service delivery. It is from these systems that specific programmes are put into operation. Each tier provides the opportunity for conceptual, structural and procedural advancement to influence post-release outcomes. It is on the basis of this model that the following recommendations will be discussed.

Prisoner outcomes are increasingly being pursued in recognition that social context influences criminal recidivism and that prisoner health has implications for public health. In this respect, the orientation of correctional philosophy has shifted, with an appreciation that effective prison management extends beyond the discrete physical and temporal boundaries of the prison sentence. To this end, many criminal justice systems are embracing prisoner rehabilitation and social reintegration interventions pre- and post-release (see, for example, Stöver (2001), which examines prison drug policy and practice in the European Union). With reference to prisoner health, the duty of care rests with prison authorities, such that (to the extent possible) the provision of health care services is adequate and deaths in custody are duly investigated. However, there exists a gap in clinical management and responsibility for ex-prisoners (Darke, 2008) and for those serving community correction orders (Biles, Harding & Walker, 1999).

The legality of duty of care for this population group is complex. Nevertheless, the concepts of prisoner health and post-release outcomes need to be broadened at the national and institutional level to ensure that the inherent right of ex-prisoners to the adequate provision of health care is upheld. This implies reframing the parameters in prison health mandates and prison outcome literature to incorporate post-discharge mortality and assigning responsibility for post-release drug treatment and management to an accountable body.

System-wide policy guidelines provide a strategic framework for consistent service delivery of drug treatment to prison populations. This facilitates the development and maintenance of the comprehensive structural processes necessary for uninterrupted professional health care throughout the criminal justice system and the subsequent amalgamation with community interventions. Such continuity of care is of particular relevance to drug dependent prisoners, who require sustained long-term treatment and case management for their chronic disorder to prevent a fatal overdose. National and regional heterogeneity of drug treatment policy and practice is, however, evident within many prison jurisdictions (Stöver, Casselman & Hennebel, 2006; Weilandt et al., 2008), which negatively affects the continuity of care.

Both political will and top-down programme coordination are essential to continuity of care. Incorporating formalized integrated multi-agency partnerships and networks among relevant prison-based and external stakeholders ensures the viability of throughcare. Also, multifaceted individualized treatment modalities that are responsive to prisoner needs promote a culture of active participation and empowerment through involvement in designing treatment plans and service options. Effective system-wide policy and practice also includes prisoner education, staff training and built-in regulatory mechanisms. The latter are necessary for identifying implementation and treatment gaps, and evaluating processes and outcomes in a continuous feedback loop.

Innovative approaches to programme delivery, especially those that facilitate familial or community interactions, can contribute to pre-release preparation. Overdose prevention programmes are of value in educating prisoners and their family members about the risks associated with reduced tolerance and the use of concomitant psychotropic substances. This prevention strategy entails teaching participants to recognize and respond to overdose symptoms (Home Office, 2009).

Naloxone, which binds preferentially to opioid receptors to counter the central nervous system and respiratory depression of an opioid overdose, has been recommended for released prisoners (Strang et al., 1996; Singleton et al., 2003; Darke, 2008). Community pilot programmes of take-home naloxone have had positive results (Dettmer, Saunders & Strang, 2001; Galea et al., 2006). Although, naloxone is provided in all Australian prison jurisdictions, formal evaluations have not been undertaken (Black, Dolan & Wodak, 2004).

Models and interventions in countries

Specific models and interventions have been developed in many countries, and examples from Australia, Canada, England and Wales, and Spain are described below.

With reference to system-wide policy and practice modalities, a case in point is that of the framework for England and Wales, which delivers an integrated multi-entry-point throughcare model of drug treatment. This national framework, the Integrated Drug Treatment System in Prisons in partnership with the Drug Interventions Programme, enlists the multidisciplinary collaboration of therapeutic jurisprudence structures. The provision of prison health care services, under the direction of the National Health Service since 2004, utilizes evidence-based therapy and, in so doing, has vastly expanded the prison-based methadone maintenance treatment programme (NHS, 2007; Weilandt et al., 2008). The objective of the Drug Interventions Programme is to guide adult drug misusers into treatment and away from crime. The commitment of political and professional entities endorses the principle of equivalence of care with community-based interventions in terms of quality, coverage and treatment alternatives. To this end, comprehensive training packages and guides (WHO Collaborating Centre for Research and Training for Mental Health et al., 2002; Weilandt et al., 2008) and protocols on modes of clinical management (DH et al., 1999, 2007; DH, 2006) have been developed for working with drug-using prisoners.

Additionally, judicial provisions – such as conditional cautioning, restrictions on bail, drug treatment and testing orders, and the drug rehabilitation requirement of community orders – redirect prisoners into treatment at the expense of the prison (NHS, 2007; Skodbo et al., 2007). The national framework also documents end-to-end strategic guidelines for throughcare and after-care, from a prisoner's first contact with the criminal justice system (DH, 2007). Indeed, team case management maintains continuity of care as individuals make the transition between prison (counselling, assessment, referral, advice and throughcare services) and the community (criminal justice integrated teams), utilizing a common data-gathering instrument, the Drug Interventions Record (NHS, 2007).

Best practice in system-wide service delivery for drug dependent prisoners requires a range of treatment options founded on evidence-based practices. This requires that interventions incorporate flexible client-centred programmes, utilizing a multiphase interdisciplinary approach of an equivalent standard to community interventions. The

WHO Regional Office for Europe (2005) has outlined harm reduction strategies of relevance to prison populations. These include needle and syringe exchange programmes, educational measures in the form of overdose prevention programmes, formalized information dissemination, outlining of treatment expectations and peer-based support, and pharmacotherapy. The Regional Office further advocates the inclusion of substitution therapy as a central component of prison pharmacotherapy interventions, in recognition of it currently being the most effective treatment to curb mortality among heroin-dependent injecting drug users (Møller et al., 2007).

Psychotherapy and psychosocial interventions are fundamental components of drug therapy and necessitate programme integrity, responsiveness to criminogenic and psychosocial needs and after-care (Stöver, 2001). Consolidating psychosocial support and pharmacotherapy is positively correlated with greater prisoner motivation to address drug-related problems (Stöver, Casselman & Hennebel, 2006). Also, in recognition that the post-liberation transition represents a period of uncertainty for many ex-prisoners, pre- and post-release programmes need to target the development of psychosocial skills and resilience as well as to provide the necessary practical support. Standardized risk assessments and screening are warranted to identify prisoners at a heightened risk of drug-related mortality. Thus, equality of care requires an integrated system-wide psychosocial and pharmacotherapeutic interface that addresses the specific post-release needs of prisoners.

Spain has the most extensive and developed prison-based harm reduction measures in Europe (WHO Regional Office for Europe, 2005; Cook & Kanaef, 2008). Over a fifth (22%) of substitution therapy in Spain is delivered in prisons, accounting for 19 010 opioid-dependent prisoners and a coverage rate of 82% (Weilandt et al., 2008). The health of prisoners in Spain is collaboratively administered by the Ministry of Health and the Ministry of Interior, which offer considerable service and treatment options. These include pre-release education (Weilandt et al., 2008) and post-release treatment referral to community services (Stöver, 2001). The utility of service delivery to drug-dependent prisoners in Spain is advanced by psychosocial interventions, which are viewed as indispensable to treatment. One criticism, however, is the restricted availability of psychosocial support (Stöver, Hennebel & Casselman, 2004; Stöver, Casselman & Hennebel, 2006; Weilandt et al., 2008) and of interventions delivered by external non-government organizations (UNAD, 2008). The latter, when present, assist post-release social re-integration.

Specific programmes may be tailored to redress the dynamic adverse health risks encountered by drug-dependent prisoners post-release by targeting the differential needs of this subpopulation. Interventions may be multimodal, incorporating such elements as skill development and problem solving, deinstitutionalization, domestic and financial management, and counselling. In this manner, the drug problem may be put in context, so as to develop an integrated care model and shift the focus from offending behaviour to building capacity. Best practice in programme development and delivery thus involves the creation of partnerships and effective working relationships with all stakeholders, including correctional and treatment staff, prisoners and external service providers.

One such initiative is the Bolwara House Transitional Centre in New South Wales, Australia, an intensive community-based pre-release programme for women with a history of drug addiction. This non-custodial therapeutic community provides structured transitional support that implements throughcare principles. It incorporates pharmacotherapy, psychosocial development and family and community reintegration in a holistic client-centred approach. The programme consists of two phases, beginning with a four-week in-house deinstitutionalization process, after which time women commence community programmes based on their assessed needs (NSW Department of Corrective Services, 2005). Such programmes include paid or voluntary employment, accommodation, parenting and education. This fosters social inclusion and rehabilitation while strengthening competences, personal resources and self-esteem.

Similarly, the Aboriginal Offender Substance Abuse Program in Canada is a national intervention that helps aboriginal men holistically address their drug dependence and offending behaviour. This programme includes substitution therapy and examines substance abuse in terms of interpersonal and transgenerational trauma. Traditional techniques, such as cultural healing practices and re-establishing spiritual connectedness, are applied in conjunction with current therapeutic measures, including risk management and skill development (Varis, McGowan & Mullins, 2006). In this way, the Program confronts the causes of aboriginal drug addiction by implementing culturally appropriate strategies.

Conclusion

In conclusion, custodial populations have markedly elevated rates of acute drug-related mortality in the period immediately after release. This is a consequence of diminished tolerance and use of multiple drugs. Nevertheless, these deaths are preventable. A number of prevention and harm reduction responses may be suitably applied at all levels of the criminal justice system.

References

Auriacombe M et al. (2004). French field experience with buprenorphine. *American Journal on Addictions*, 13(Suppl. 1):S17–S28.

Betteridge G (2005). *Harm reduction in prisons and jails: international experience.* Toronto, Canadian HIV/AIDS Legal Network (http://www.aidslaw.ca/publications/interfaces/downloadFile.php?ref=158, accessed 5 March 2010).

Biles D, Harding R, Walker J (1999). *The deaths of offenders serving community corrections orders.* Canberra, Australian Institute of Criminology (Trends and Issues in Crime and Criminal Justice Series, No. 107; http://www.aic.gov.au/ documents/E/A/7/%7BEA798A1D-7045-4F38-AD11-8EEF8CD69B16%7Dti107.pdf, accessed 17 February 2010).

Binswanger IA et al. (2007). Release from prison – a high risk of death for former inmates. *New England Journal of Medicine*, 356:157–165.

Bird SM, Hutchinson SJ (2003). Male drugs-related deaths in the fortnight after release from prison: Scotland, 1996–99. *Addiction*, 98:185–190.

Black E, Dolan K, Wodak A (2004). *Supply, demand and harm reduction strategies in Australian prisons: implementation, cost and evaluation.* Canberra, Australian National Council on Drugs (ANCD Research Paper No. 9; http://www.ancd.org.au/images/PDF/Researchpapers/rp9_australian_prisons.pdf, accessed 17 February 2010).

Borzycki M (2005). *Interventions for prisoners returning to the community.* Canberra, Attorney-General's Department (http://www.crimeprevention.gov.au/agd/WWW/ncphome.nsf/AllDocs/DAD69C1C8D3D5F28CA256FDB001DD4B4?OpenDocument, accessed 17 February 2010).

Caplehorn JR et al. (1996). Methadone maintenance and addicts' risk of fatal heroin overdose. *Substance Use & Misuse*, 31:177–196.

Christensen PB et al. (2006). Mortality among Danish drug users released from prison. *International Journal of Prisoner Health*, 2:13–19.

Coffey C et al. (2003). Mortality in young offenders: retrospective cohort study. *British Medical Journal*, 326:1064–1066.

CE Committee of Ministers (1998). *Recommendation No. R 98(7) of the Committee of Ministers to Member States concerning the ethical and organisational aspects of health care in prison.* Strasbourg, Committee of Ministers of the Council of Europe (https://wcd.coe.int/com.instranet.InstraServlet?command=com.instranet.CmdBlobGet&InstranetImage=530914&SecMode=1&DocId=463258&Usage=2, accessed 17 February 2010).

CE Committee of Ministers (2006). *Recommendation No. R 06(2) of the Committee of Ministers to member states concerning the European prison rules.* Strasbourg,

Committee of Ministers of the Council of Europe (https://wcd.coe.int/ViewDoc.jsp?id=955747, accessed 17 February 2010).

Cook C, Kanaef N (2008). *The global state of harm reduction 2008: mapping the response to drug-related HIV and hepatitis C epidemics*. London, International Harm Reduction Association (http://www.ihra.net/GlobalState2008, accessed 17 February 2008).

Crowley D (1999). The drug detox unit at Mountjoy prison – a review. *Journal of Health Gain*, 3:17–19.

Cushman P Jr (1977). Ten years of methadone maintenance treatment: some clinical observations. *American Journal of Drug and Alcohol Abuse*, 4:543–553.

Darke S (2008). From the can to the coffin: deaths among recently released prisoners. *Addiction*, 103:256–257.

Darke S, Zador D (1996). Fatal heroin 'overdose': a review. *Addiction*, 91, 1765–1772.

Davies S, Cook S (2000). *Dying outside: women, imprisonment and post-release mortality. Women in Corrections: Staff and Clients Conference, Adelaide, Australia, 31 October – 1 November 2000*. Griffith, Australian Institute of Criminology (http://www.aic.gov.au/events/aic%20upcoming%20events/2000/~/media/conferences/womencorrections/cookdavi.ashx, accessed 5 March 2010).

Davoli M et al. (1993). Risk factors for overdose mortality: a case-control study within a cohort of intravenous drug users. *International Journal of Epidemiology*, 22:273–277.

Dettmer K, Saunders B, Strang J (2001). Take home naloxone and the prevention of deaths from opiate overdose: two pilot schemes. *British Medical Journal*, 322, 895–896.

DH (2006). *Clinical management of drug dependence in the adult prison setting: including psychosocial treatment as a core part*. London, Department of Health (England) (http://www.nta.nhs.uk/publications/documents/clinical_management_of_drug_dependence_in_the_adult_prison_setting.pdf, accessed 17 February 2010).

DH (2007). *Prisons integrated drug treatment system: continuity of care guidance*. London, Department of Health (England) (http://www.nta.nhs.uk/areas/criminal_justice/docs/continuity_of_care_guidance.doc, accessed 17 February 2010).

DH et al. (1999). *Drug misuse and dependence – guidelines on clinical management*. London, Her Majesty's Stationary Office (http://www.dh.gov.uk/prod_consum_dh/groups/dh_digitalassets/@dh/@en/documents/digitalasset/dh_4078198.pdf, accessed 17 February 2010).

DH et al. (2007). *Drug misuse and dependence – UK guidelines on clinical management*. London, Department of Health (England), the Scottish Government,

Welsh Assembly Government and Northern Ireland Executive (http://www.nta.nhs.uk/publications/documents/clinical_guidelines_2007.pdf, accessed 5 March).

Dolan KA et al. (2005). Four-year follow-up of imprisoned male heroin users and methadone treatment: mortality, re-incarceration and hepatitis C infection. *Addiction*, 100:820–828.

EMCDDA (2008). *Statistical bulletin 2008*. Lisbon, European Monitoring Centre for Drugs and Drug Addiction (http://www.emcdda.europa.eu/stats08, accessed 17 February 2010).

Farrell M, Marsden J (2005). *Drug-related mortality among newly-released offenders 1998 to 2000*. London, Home Office (Home Office Online Report 40/05; http://www.drugscope.org.uk/OneStopCMS/Core/CrawlerResourceServer.aspx?resource=27ECC17D-CEF3-451E-8DBB-4336FA695ECB&mode=link&guid=c460f97af5e449f189088a5545d9175c, accessed 17 February 2010).

Farrell M, Marsden J (2008). Acute risk of drug-related death among newly released prisoners in England and Wales. *Addiction*, 103:251–255.

Fazel S, Bains P, Doll H (2006). Substance abuse and dependence in prisoners: a systematic review. *Addiction*, 101:181–191.

Fox A et al. (2005). *Throughcare and aftercare: approaches and promising practice in service delivery for clients released from prison or leaving residential rehabilitation*. London, Home Office (Online Report 01/05; http://www.homeoffice.gov.uk/rds/pdfs05/rdsolr0105.pdf, accessed 5 March 2010).

Galea S et al. (2006). Provision of naloxone to injection drug users as an overdose prevention strategy: early evidence from a pilot study in New York City. *Addictive Behaviors*, 31:907–912.

Gearing FR, Schweitzer MD (1974). An epidemiologic evaluation of long-term methadone maintenance treatment for heroin addiction. *American Journal of Epidemiology*, 100:101–112.

Gossop M et al. (2002). A prospective study of mortality among drug misusers during a 4-year period after seeking treatment. *Addiction*, 97:39–47.

Graham A (2003). Post-prison mortality: unnatural death among people released from Victorian prisons between January 1990 and December 1999. *Australian and New Zealand Journal of Criminology*, 36:94–108.

Grönbladh L, Ohlund LS, Gunne LM (1990). Mortality in heroin addiction: impact of methadone treatment. *Acta Psychiatrica Scandinavica*, 82:223–227.

Gunne LM, Grönbladh L (1981). The Swedish methadone maintenance program: a controlled study. *Drug and Alcohol Dependence*, 7:249–256.

Harding-Pink D (1990). Mortality following release from prison. *Medicine, Science and the Law*, 30:12–16.

Hobbs M et al. (2006). *Mortality and morbidity in prisoners after release from prison in Western Australia 1995–2003.* Canberra, Australian Institute of Criminology (Trends and Issues in Crime and Criminal Justice Series, No. 320; http://www.aic.gov.au/documents/6/7/3/%7B6731BD68-AD7F-48CF-B527-2D3C4FA71E13%7Dtandi320.pdf, 7 March 2010).

Home Office (2009). *Around arrest, beyond release 2: moving forward – identifying and promoting practice to meet the needs of families in relation to the arrest and release of drug-misusing offenders.* London, Home Office (http://drugs.homeoffice.gov.uk/publication-search/dip/around-arrest-beyond-release-2/report2835.pdf?view=Binary, accessed 18 March 2010).

Kariminia A et al. (2007a). Extreme cause-specific mortality in a cohort of adult prisoners – 1988 to 2002: a data-linkage study. *International Journal of Epidemiology*, 36:310–316.

Kariminia A et al. (2007b). Factors associated with mortality in a cohort of Australian prisoners. *European Journal of Epidemiology*, 22:417–428.

Kariminia A et al. (2007c). Suicide risk among recently released prisoners in New South Wales, Australia. *Medical Journal of Australia*, 187:387–390.

Kastelic A, Pont J, Stöver H (2008). *Opioid substitution treatment in custodial settings: a practical guide.* Oldenburg, BIS-Verlag der Carl von Ossietzky Universität Oldenburg.

Langendam MW et al. (2001). The impact of harm-reduction-based methadone treatment on mortality among heroin users. *American Journal of Public Health*, 91:774–780.

Lines R et al. (2004). *Dublin declaration on HIV/AIDS in prisons in Europe and Central Asia: good prison health is good public health.* Dublin, Irish Penal Reform Trust (http://www.penalreform.org/resources/rep-2004-dublin-declaration-en.pdf, accessed 18 February 2010).

McGregor C et al. (1999). *It's rarely just the 'h': addressing overdose among South Australian heroin users through a process of intersectoral collaboration.* Parkside, Drug and Alcohol Services Council of South Australia (http://www.drugpolicy.org/docUploads/mcgregor2.pdf, accessed 18 February 2010).

Møller L et al., eds (2007). *Health in prisons: a WHO guide to the essentials in prison health.* Copenhagen, WHO Regional Office for Europe (http://www.euro.who.int/document/e90174.pdf, accessed 18 February 2010).

NSW Department of Corrective Services (2005). *Inmate classification and placement procedures manual.* Sydney, NSW Department of Corrective Services (http://www.nswccl.org.au/docs/dcs/CLASSMAN_UPD%202005%20DRAFT%204%20-%20interim.doc, accessed 18 February 2010).

NHS (2007). *Key messages for the drug interventions programme – February 2007.* London, National Treatment Agency for Substance Misuse (http://www.nta.nhs.uk/areas/criminal_justice/docs/ho_dip_key_mes_feb07.pdf, accessed 18 February 2010).

Poser W, Koc J, Ehrenreich H (1995). Methadone maintenance treatment. Methadone treatment can reduce mortality. *British Medical Journal*, 310:463.

Sattar G (2001). *Rates and causes of death among prisoners and offenders under community supervision.* London, Home Office (Home Office Research Study 231; http://www.homeoffice.gov.uk/rds/pdfs/hors231.pdf, 18 February 2010).

Seal KH et al. (2001). Predictors and prevention of nonfatal overdose among street-recruited injection heroin users in the San Francisco Bay Area, 1998–1999. *American Journal of Public Health*, 91:1842–1846.

Seaman SR, Brettle RP, Gore SM (1998). Mortality from overdose among injecting drug users recently released from prison: database linkage study. *British Medical Journal*, 316:426–428.

Seymour A, Oliver JS, Black M (2000). Drug-related deaths among recently released prisoners in the Strathclyde Region of Scotland. *Journal of Forensic Sciences*, 45:649–654.

Shewan D et al. (2000). Fatal drug overdose after liberation from prison: a retrospective study of female ex-prisoners from Strathclyde Region (Scotland). *Addiction Research and Theory*, 8:267–278.

Shewan D et al. (2001). Injecting risk behaviour among recently released prisoners in Edinburgh: the impact of in-prison and community drug treatment services. *Legal and Criminological Psychology*, 6:19–28.

Singleton N et al. (2003). *Drug-related mortality among newly released offenders.* London, Home Office (Home Office Online Report 16/03; http://www.homeoffice.gov.uk/rds/pdfs2/rdsolr1603.pdf, accessed 18 February 2010).

Skodbo S et al. (2007). *The drug interventions programme (DIP): addressing drug use and offending through 'Tough Choices'.* London, Home Office (http://www.homeoffice.gov.uk/rds/pdfs07/horr02c.pdf, accessed 18 February 2010).

Stewart LM et al. (2004). Risk of death in prisoners after release from jail. *Australian and New Zealand Journal of Public Health*, 28:32–36.

Stöver H (2001). *Assistance to drug users in European Union prisons: an overview study.* London, European Network for Drug and HIV/AIDS Services in Prison and European Monitoring Centre for Drugs and Drug Addiction.

Stöver H, Casselman J, Hennebel L (2006). Substitution treatment in European prisons: a study of policies and practices in 18 European countries. *International Journal of Prisoner Health*, 2:3–12.

Stöver H, Hennebel LC, Casselman J. (2004). *Substitution treatment in European prisons: a study of policies and practices of substitution in prisons in 18 European countries*. London, European Network of Drug Services in Prison.

Strang J et al. (1996). Heroin overdose: the case for take-home naloxone. *British Medical Journal*, 312:1435–1436.

United Nations (1946). Constitution of the World Health Organization. *Official Records of the World Health Organization*, 2:100 (http://www.who.int/governance/eb/who_constitution_en.pdf, accessed 5 March 2010).

United Nations (1948). *The Universal Declaration of Human Rights*. New York, United Nations (http://www.un.org/en/documents/udhr/, accessed 18 February 2010): Article 25.

United Nations (1955). *Standard Minimum Rules for the Treatment of Prisoners: adopted by the First United Nations Congress on the Prevention of Crime and the Treatment of Offenders on 30 August 1955, UN Doc A/CONF/611, Annex I, ESC Res 663C, 24 UN ESCOR Supp (No 1) at 11, UN Doc E/3048 (1957), amended by ESC Res 2076, 62 UN ESCOR Supp (No 1) at 35, UN Doc E/5988 (1977)*. New York, United Nations (http://www1.umn.edu/humanrts/instree/g1smr.htm, accessed 5 March 2010).

United Nations (1976a). *International Covenant on Civil and Political Rights*. Geneva, Office of the High Commissioner for Human Rights. (http://www2.ohchr.org/english/law/ccpr.htm, accessed 18 February 2008): Articles 6–7.

United Nations (1976b). *International Covenant on Economic, Social, and Cultural Rights*. Geneva, Office of the High Commissioner for Human Rights (http://www2.ohchr.org/english/law/cescr.htm, accessed 18 February 2008): Article 12.

United Nations (1982). *Principles of medical ethics*. New York, United Nations (document A/RES/37/194; http://www.un.org/documents/ga/res/37/a37r194.htm, accessed 18 February 2010).

United Nations (1988). *Body of principles for the protection of all persons under any form of detention or imprisonment*. New York, United Nations (document A/RES/43/173; http://www.un.org/documents/ga/res/43/a43r173.htm, accessed 5 March 2010).

United Nations (1990). *Basic principles for the treatment of prisoners: annex*. New York, United Nations (document A/Res 45/111; http://www.un.org/documents/ga/res/45/a45r111.htm, accessed 5 March 2010).

UNODC, UNAIDS, WHO (2006). *HIV/AIDS prevention, care, treatment and support in prison settings: a framework for an efficient national response.* Vienna, United Nations Office on Drugs and Crime (http://www.unodc.org/documents/hiv-aids/HIV-AIDS_prisons_Oct06.pdf, accessed 18 February 2010).

Varis DD, McGowan V, Mullins P (2006). Development of an Aboriginal Offender Substance Abuse Program. *FORUM on Corrections Research*, 18:42–44 (http://www.csc-scc.gc.ca/text/pblct/forum/e181/e181j_e.pdf, accessed 18 February 2010).

Verger P et al. (2003). High mortality rates among inmates during the year following their discharge from a French prison. *Journal of Forensic Science*, 48:614–616.

Warren E et al. (2006). Value for money in drug treatment: economic evaluation of prison methadone. *Drug and Alcohol Dependence*, 84:160–166.

Weilandt C et al. (2008). *Reduction of drug-related crime in prison: the impact of opioid substitution treatment on the manageability of opioid dependent prisoners.* Bremen, Bremen Institute for Drug Research, University of Bremen; Bonn, WIAD – Scientific Institute of the German Medical Association.

WHO (1993). *WHO guidelines on HIV infection and AIDS in prisons.* Geneva, World Health Organization (http://www.who.int/hiv/idu/WHO-Guidel-Prisons_en.pdf, accessed 18 February 2010).

WHO Collaborating Centre for Research and Training for Mental Health et al. (2002). *Mental health primary care in prison: adapted for prisons and young offender institutions from the WHO guide to mental health in primary care.* London, Royal Society of Medicine Press (http://www.prisonmentalhealth.org, accessed 18 February 2010).

WHO Regional Office for Europe (2003). *Declaration on prison health as part of public health.* Copenhagen, WHO Regional Office for Europe (http://www.euro.who.int/Document/HIPP/moscow_declaration_eng04.pdf, accessed 18 February 2010).

WHO Regional Office for Europe (2005). *Status paper on prisons, drugs and harm reduction.* Copenhagen, WHO Regional Office for Europe (http://www.euro.who.int/document/e85877.pdf, accessed 18 February 2010).

WHO, UNODC, UNAIDS (2004). *Substitution maintenance therapy in the management of opioid dependence and HIV/AIDS prevention: position paper.* Geneva, World Health Organization (http://www.unodc.org/docs/treatment/Brochure_E.pdf, accessed 18 February 2010).

Zador D, Sunjic S, Darke S. (1996). Heroin-related deaths in New South Wales, 1992: toxicological findings and circumstances. *Medical Journal of Australia*, 164:204–207.